This book is dedicated to

my mom, husband, and two beautiful boys, Philip and Alex

And to my Ava Bella Day Spa family,
none of this would have come to fruition without your support

DeeDee

Introduction

Homemade remedies go back as far as one can remember. Cleopatra was known for her beautiful skin and make-up. It's noted in old text that she often bathed in lavishing milk baths, performed milk masks on her face and used coal for make-up. There's also record of Queen Nefertiti taking care of her luscious skin with natural ingredients. They knew the benefits of pampering, even back in B.C.

Fresh fruits, vegetables , plants, and herbs have shaped the beauty industry. The majority of body lotions, skin care, hair products and make-up found on the shelves are derived from perishable items.

 This book is a guide on how to take care of your skin with ingredients in your kitchen, garden, and fridge. My hope is to have your own skin care remedies, for your specific skin type, without having to spend a fortune. Take some time for yourself, pamper yourself , and reward yourself for all the hard work you do.

The benefits of taking care of your number one organ, your skin, are endless. Besides the confidence gained from having fabulous skin, you'll feel healthier. These benefits increase the longevity and quality of your life.

From anti-aging to body treatments, acne to exfoliants, this book will provide you with the recipes and tools you need to achieve your skin care goals.
Enjoy!

Table of Contents

Cleansers and Toners:

Purifying Grape Cleansers   2
Apple Toner   3
Oily Skin Tonic   4
Peaches and Cream Exfoliant Cleanser   5

Exfoliants:

At Home Microdermabrasion   7
Coffee with Cream and Sugar   8
Pumpkin Pie Peel   9
Apricot Poppy Seed Exfoliant   10
Soothing Facial Peel   11
Pineapple and Cornmeal Exfoliant   12
Strawberry Rice Daily Exfoliant   13

Treatments:

Acne Spot Treatment   15
Soothing Eye Repair   16

Masks:

Tightening Exfoliating Mask 18
Applesauce and Honey Mask 19
Banana Cream Anti- Acne Mask 20-21
Blackberry Kiwi Lightening Mask 22
Blueberry Oatmeal Mask 23
Milk and Honey Recovery Mask 24
Yogurt, Cucumber, and Green Tea Mask 25
Avocado Mango Glow 26
Sweet Potato Pomegranate Wrinkle Mask 27
Smoothie Mask 28
Kiwi Grapefruit Mask 29
Aspirin Mask 30
Tomato Garlic Lemon Mask 31

Body Treatments:

Chocolate Covered Strawberry Scrub 33
Pumpkin Pie Body Scrub 34
Café Mocha Latte Cellulite Scrub 35
Seaweed Wrap 36-37

Cleanser and Toners

It is important to cleanse your skin every day and/or night to remove make-up, impurities, dead skin cells, and excess oil. The best way to cleanse your skin is with luke warm water. Apply the cleanser to wet skin, then rinse.

Using a toner is vital to helping your skin retain it's PH balance. When your skin's PH is out of balance, you experience drier, dehydrated skin or notice excessive oil. It's best to use a toner after you cleanse your skin and before you moisturize.

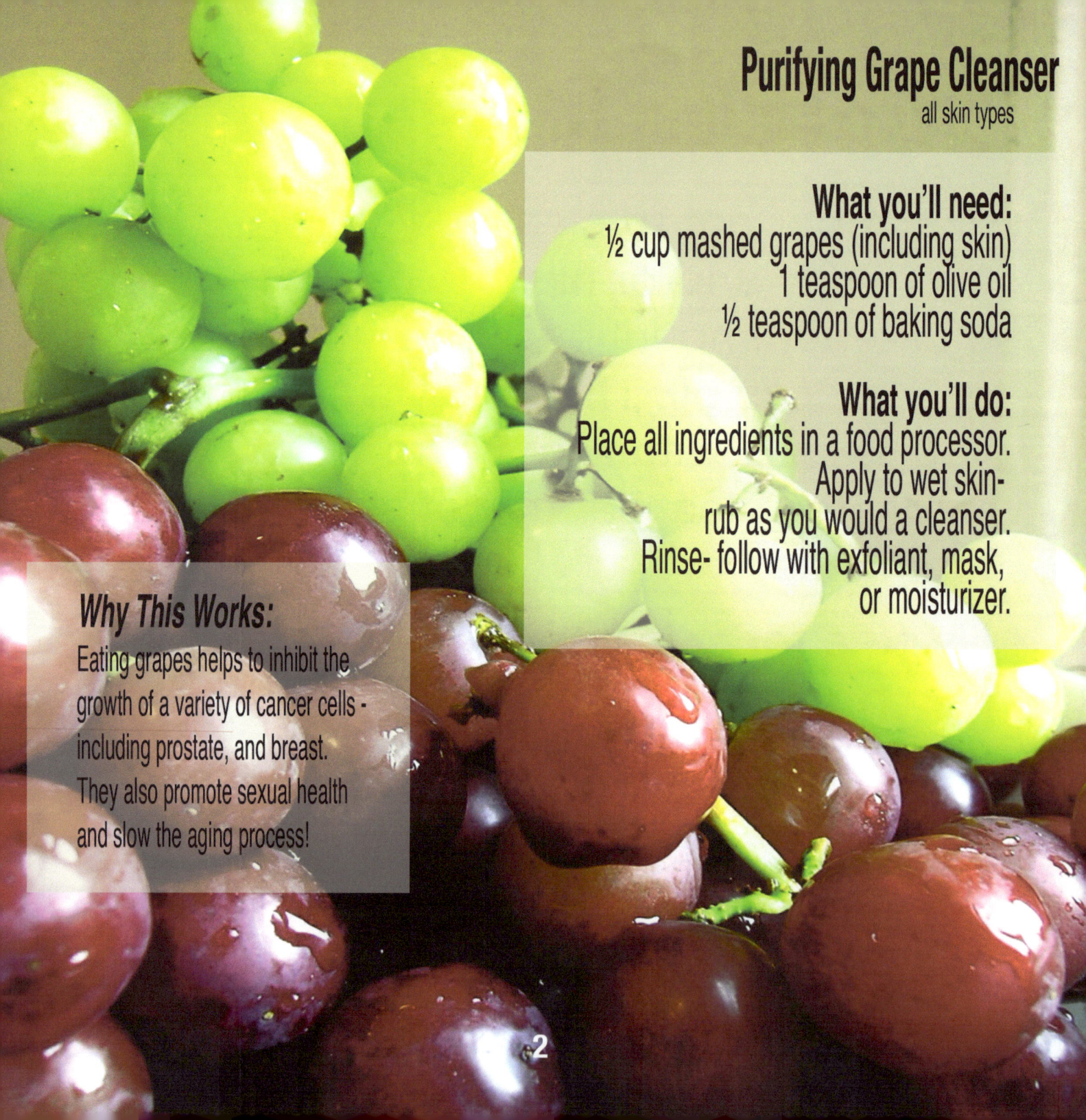

Purifying Grape Cleanser
all skin types

What you'll need:
½ cup mashed grapes (including skin)
1 teaspoon of olive oil
½ teaspoon of baking soda

What you'll do:
Place all ingredients in a food processor.
Apply to wet skin-
rub as you would a cleanser.
Rinse- follow with exfoliant, mask,
or moisturizer.

Why This Works:
Eating grapes helps to inhibit the
growth of a variety of cancer cells -
including prostate, and breast.
They also promote sexual health
and slow the aging process!

Apple Toner
all skin types

This is a beautiful toner that is safe to use throughout the day.
It helps with flakiness from dry skin and to control oily skin.
It also helps tired and stressed out skin look more vibrant.

What You'll Need:

1 granny smith or red delicious apple

What You'll Do:

Simply take the apple and juice it.
Apply the juice to your skin with a cotton ball.
No need to rinse- just follow with a moisturizer.

Oily Skin Tonic

oily skin
acne prone

What You'll Need:

1 cup of distilled water
1 Tablespoon of grated apple (any type of apple is fine)
¼ teaspoon of pepper
1 teaspoon of apple cider vinegar

What You'll Do:

First, bring distilled water to a boil.
Add all ingredients and turn off the stove.
Let sit for two hours.
Strain the liquid with a strainer and cheese cloth
 (or through a thin paper towel).
Using cotton balls or gauze- apply to cleansed face.
The excess liquid can be refrigerated for a few days.
Use as often as you like throughout the day.

Peaches and Cream Exfoliating Cleanser
all skin types

What You'll Need:
1 Tablespoon of Baking Soda
½ Peach
1 Tablespoon of Yogurt

What You'll Do:
Puree the peach (in a blender).
In a small bowl, combine yogurt and
 pureed peach.
Fold in the baking soda.
Use to cleanse your skin- rubbing in
 circular motions to exfoliate.
Rinse and apply appropriate moisturizer.

Reasons Why We Exfoliate...

Skin cells have a life of around 25 days, they then naturally shed to make room for the new skin cells. Sometimes the old skin cells remain attached to the surface of your skin, which can create challenges for the new cells.

Blackheads, whiteheads, rough texture, or an uneven appearance of the skin tone are a result.
They also suffocate the new cells- compromising the elasticity of the collagen, and causing premature wrinkles.

When the natural process of shedding the dead, dry skin cells doesn't work, you need to step in and help it along.

Keeping the skin exfoliated helps ensure the longevity of the cells, elasticity of the collagen, and helps your products to pass through deeper into the dermis. This is exactly what we want to slow down the process of aging.

At Home Microdermabrasion
all skin types

What You'll Need:
1 Tablespoon of baking soda
2 teaspoons of water

What You'll Do:
Mix the 2 ingredients to make a paste.
    In circular motions-rub the paste
    over entire face, neck, and
    décolleté using your fingertips.
You can go up to the eye area as well.
After rubbing for 2-5 minutes- rinse.
Continue doing this once a week for several weeks.
You will notice a significant difference in your skin tone.
Don't forget to wear your sunscreen!

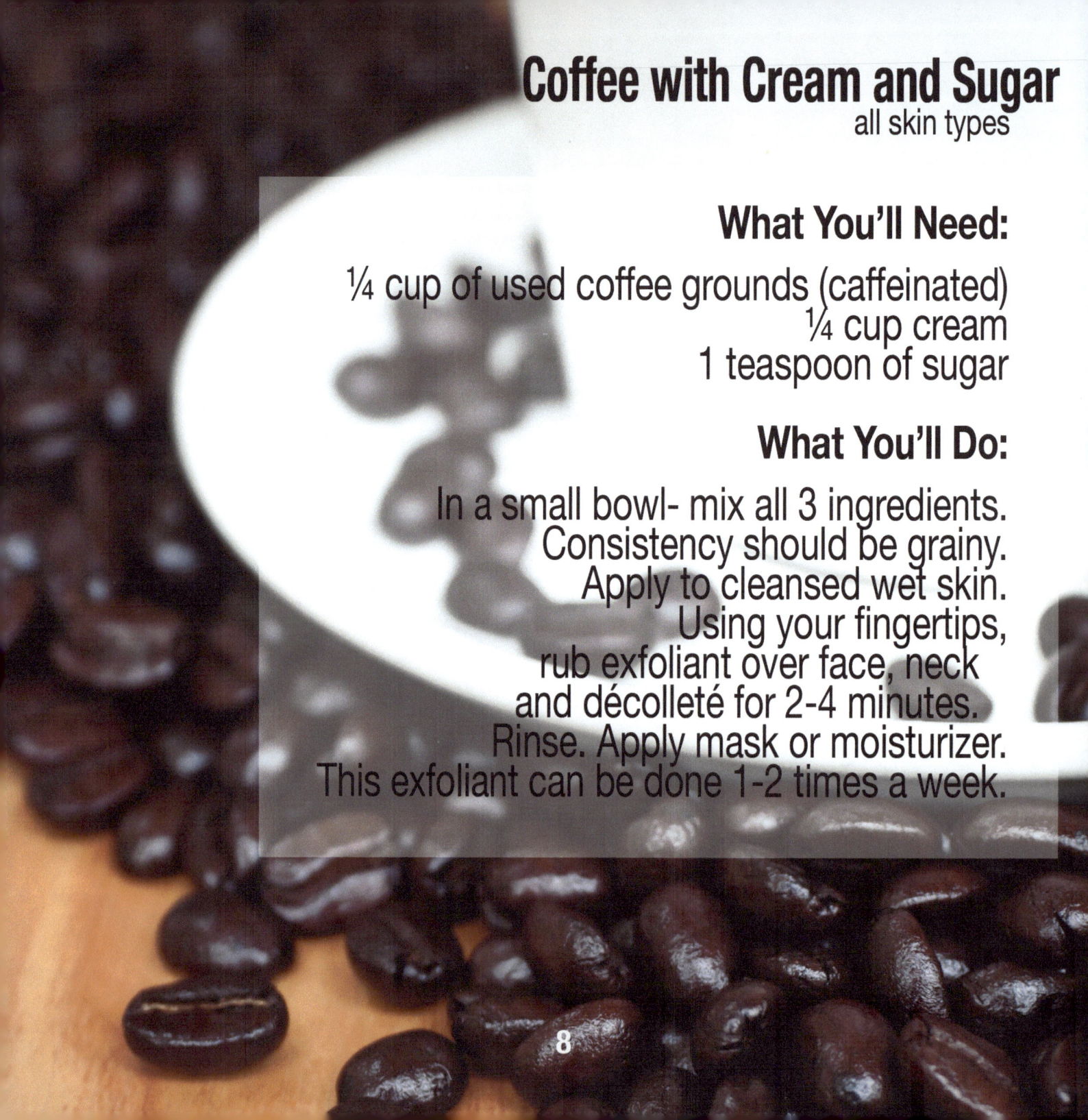

Coffee with Cream and Sugar
all skin types

What You'll Need:

¼ cup of used coffee grounds (caffeinated)
¼ cup cream
1 teaspoon of sugar

What You'll Do:

In a small bowl- mix all 3 ingredients.
Consistency should be grainy.
Apply to cleansed wet skin.
Using your fingertips,
rub exfoliant over face, neck
and décolleté for 2-4 minutes.
Rinse. Apply mask or moisturizer.
This exfoliant can be done 1-2 times a week.

Pumpkin Pie Peel

oily
acne prone
anti- aging

What You'll Need:

¼ cup of mashed pumpkin (may be canned)
1 Tablespoon of cream
1 teaspoon of cinnamon

What You'll Do:

*This is a very strong peel.
If you feel an uncomfortable
burning of the skin,
remove immediately.*

In a small bowl, mix together all ingredients.
Apply to cleansed skin for 5 minutes.
Remove and follow with appropriate
moisturizer and sunscreen.

Do not forget your sunscreen,
your skin will b extra sensitive to the sun
following the peel.

Apricot Poppy Seed Exfoliant
all skin types

What You'll Need:

1 teaspoon of poppy seeds
¼ cup mashed apricots
1 teaspoon of honey

What You'll Do:

Mix all ingredients together.
Apply to cleansed skin.
Rub in circular motions,
 around entire face, neck and chest.
Don't forget eye area.
Remove and apply moisturizer.

Spa Tip-

It's essential to exfoliate your skin. Removing of the dead skin cells will decrease the aging process. It's recommended to exfoliate 2-3 times a week.

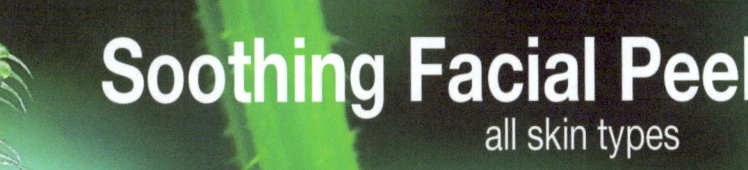

Soothing Facial Peel
all skin types

What You'll Need:

1 teaspoon of mashed cucumber
½ teaspoon of honey
½ teaspoon of sour cream

What You'll Do:

In a small bowl, mix the three ingredients together.
Apply to cleansed face, neck, and décolleté
Leave on for 10 minutes.
Rinse and apply appropriate mask or moisturizer

11

Pineapple and Cornmeal Exfoliant

all skin types

What You'll Need:

½ cup of pineapple
¼ cup of cornmeal
1 Tablespoon of olive oil

What You'll Do:

First, blend or purée the pineapple
   to a semi-smooth consistency.
Then mix the cornmeal
   and the olive oil with the pineapple.
On cleansed wet skin,
   rub in circular motions
   over face, neck, and décolleté.
Do this for a couple of minutes.
Rinse and apply appropriate moisturizer
   and sunscreen.

Strawberry Rice Exfoliant

This is a daily exfoliant.
It can be used on acne prone, to even the most sensitive skin.

What You'll Need:

¼ cup mashed strawberries
1 Tablespoon of rice powder
   (ground uncooked rice in a food processor until
   consistency is of a fine powder).
Use either brown or white rice.

What You'll Do:

Mix both ingredients together.
Apply to cleansed, damp skin.
Rub over entire face, neck, and décolleté.
Rinse.
Follow with mask or moisturizer.

Did You Know?

Strawberries help to decrease the craving of nicotine? So- not only will they exfoliate your skin, they'll also help kick the habit!

Treatments

These recipes are "add on" recipes for your skin. They are designed to give your skin an extra boost in certain areas. These treatments are in addition to your regular skin care regimen. It's okay to do these as often as you like. Try adding one to a mask and see if you notice a difference.

Have fun with them!

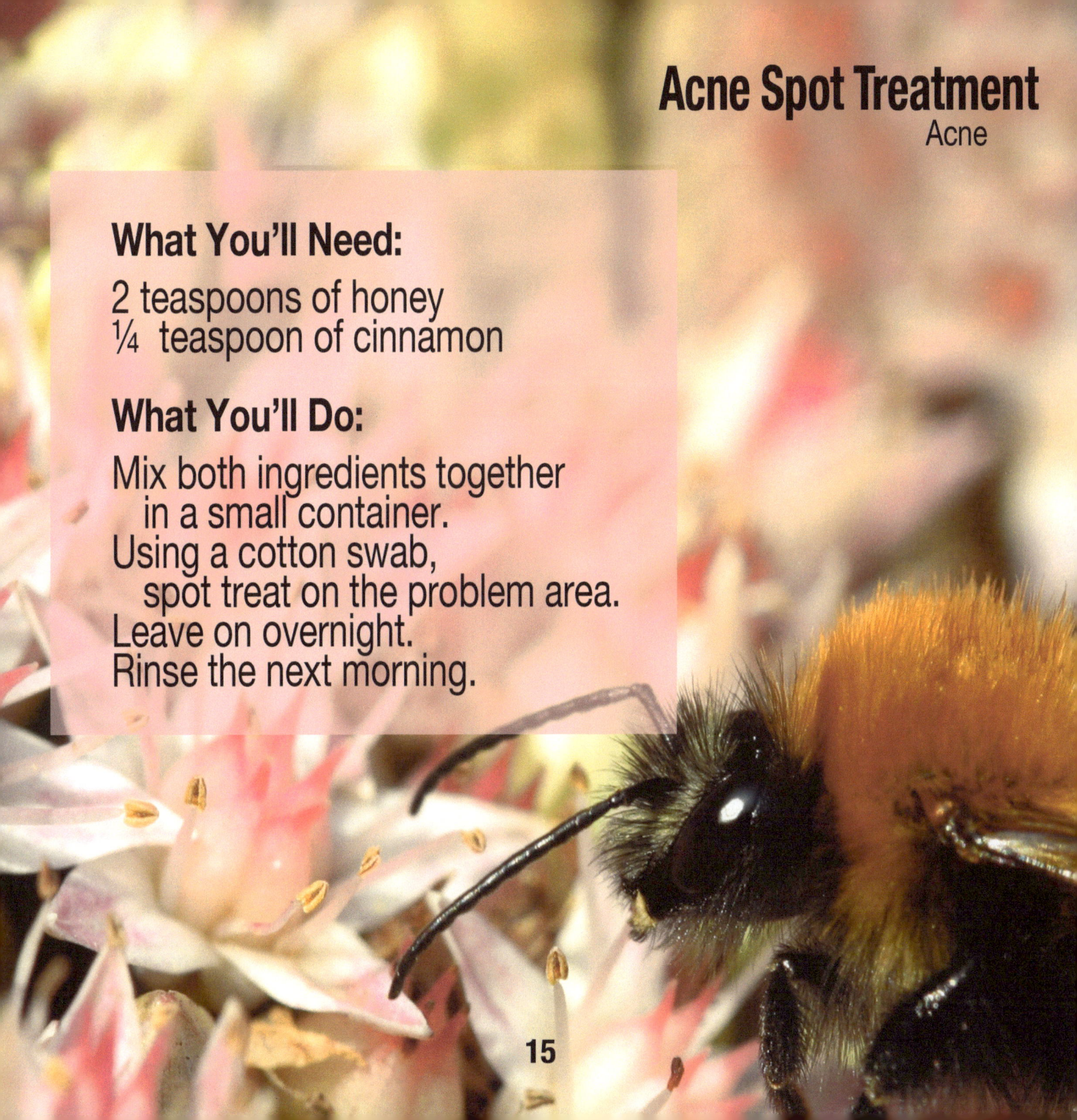

What You'll Need:

2 teaspoons of honey
¼ teaspoon of cinnamon

What You'll Do:

Mix both ingredients together
   in a small container.
Using a cotton swab,
   spot treat on the problem area.
Leave on overnight.
Rinse the next morning.

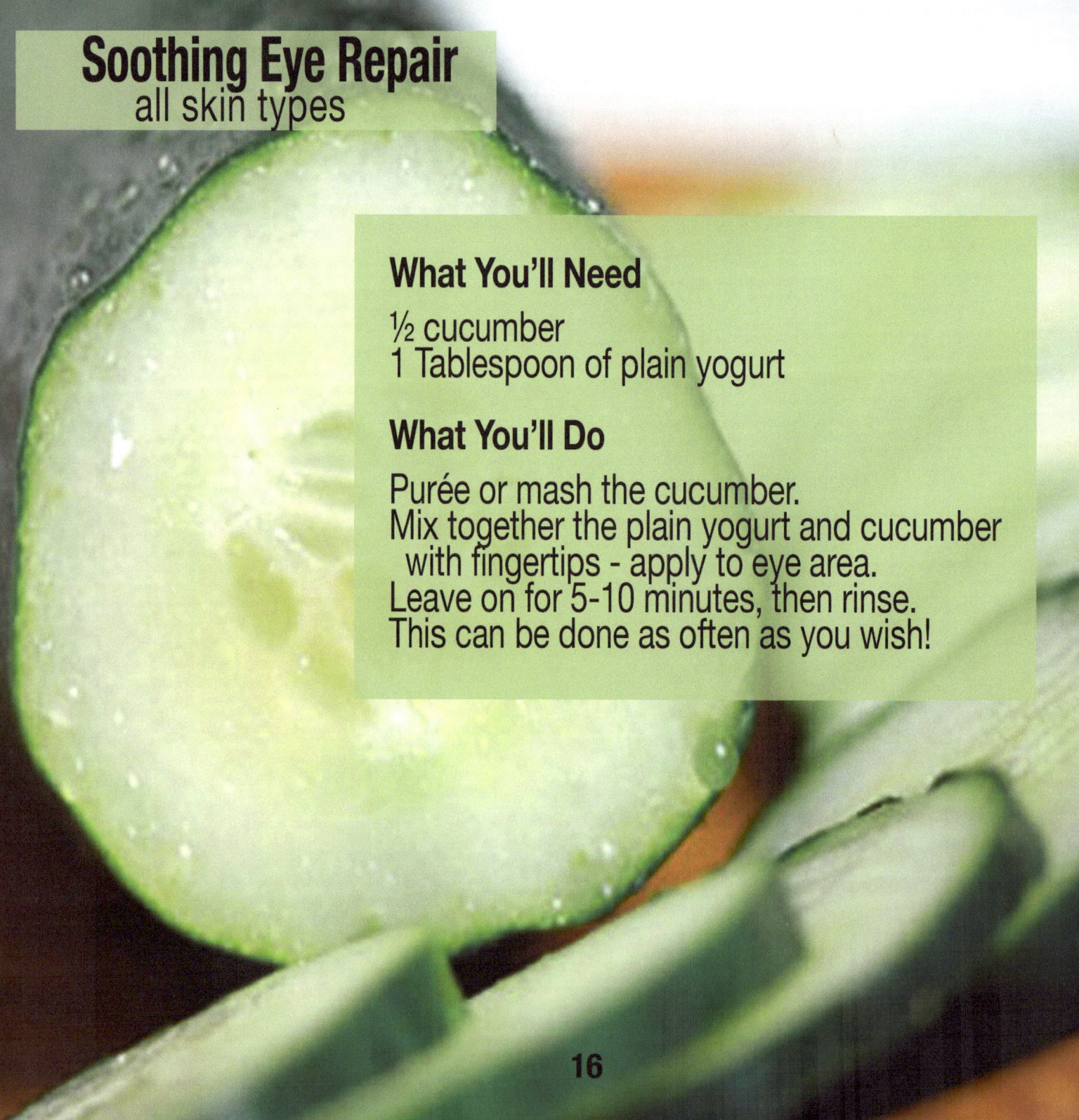

Soothing Eye Repair
all skin types

What You'll Need

½ cucumber
1 Tablespoon of plain yogurt

What You'll Do

Purée or mash the cucumber.
Mix together the plain yogurt and cucumber
 with fingertips - apply to eye area.
Leave on for 5-10 minutes, then rinse.
This can be done as often as you wish!

Why Mask?

A facial mask is intended to treat certain skin conditions. Whether your concerns are hydration, acne, oil control, or anti-aging, a mask is a great way to nourish your skin.

Some of the benefits of masking include:
- tighten and tone
- decrease pore size
- hydrate
- calm and soothe
- control acne

The best time to use a mask is after cleansing and exfoliating. Try using them a couple times a week. Experiment with the different masks. See if you notice a difference.
Don't forget to apply to your neck and chest!

Tightening Exfoliating Mask
all skin types

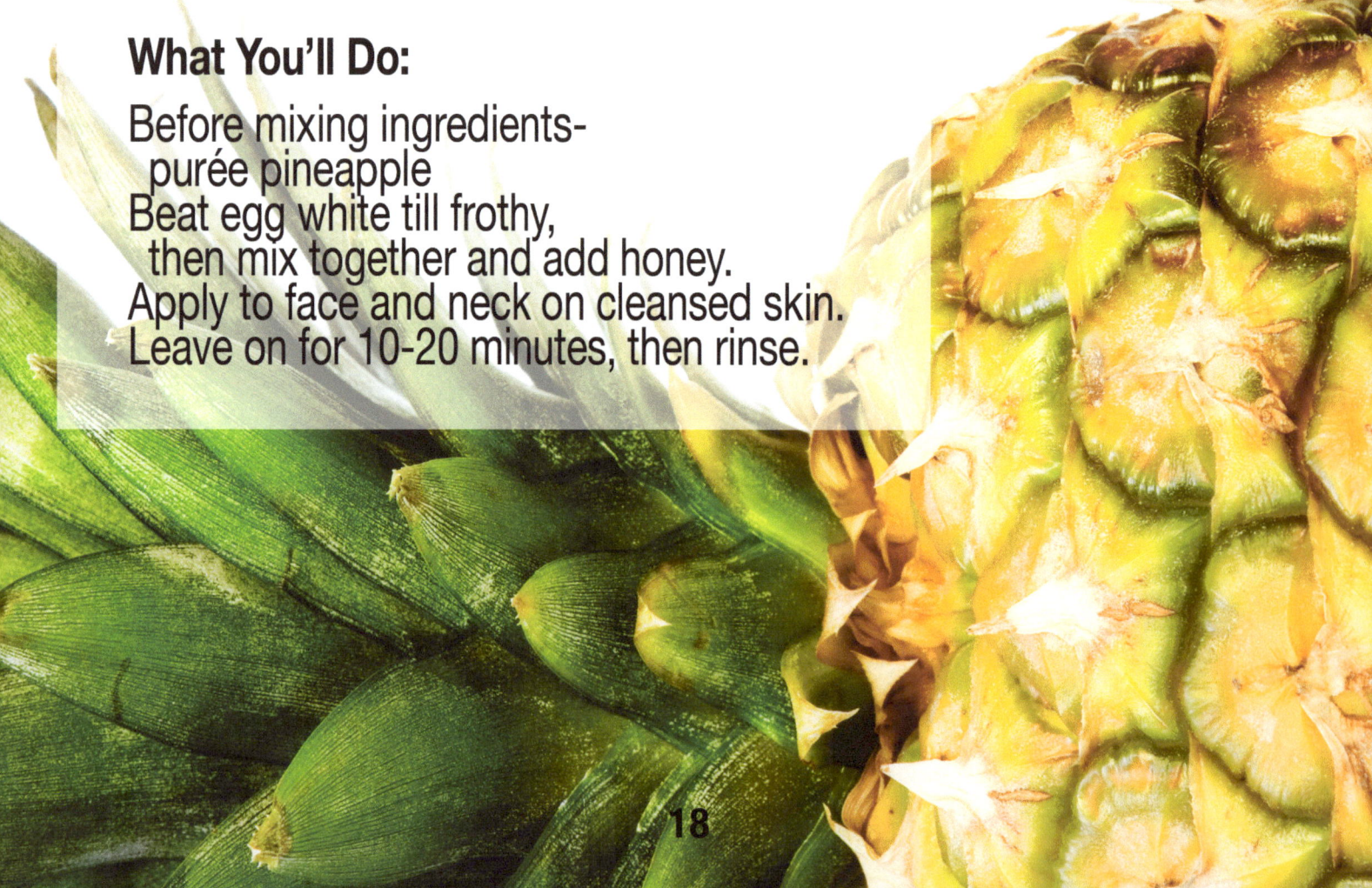

What You'll Need:

¼ cup pineapple chunks
1 egg white
1 teaspoon of honey

What You'll Do:

Before mixing ingredients-
 purée pineapple
Beat egg white till frothy,
 then mix together and add honey.
Apply to face and neck on cleansed skin.
Leave on for 10-20 minutes, then rinse.

18

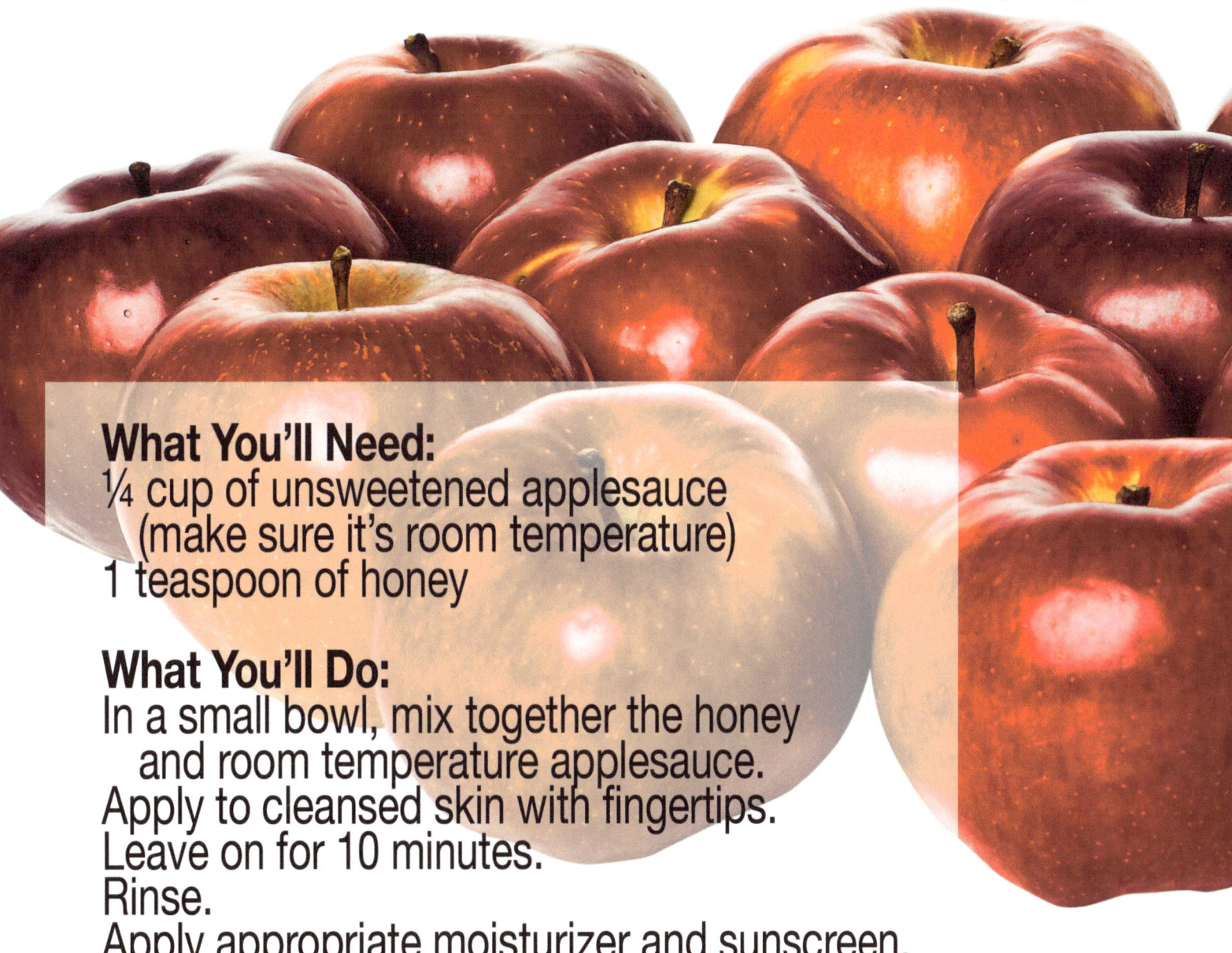

Applesauce and Honey Mask
sensitive skin

What You'll Need:
¼ cup of unsweetened applesauce
   (make sure it's room temperature)
1 teaspoon of honey

What You'll Do:
In a small bowl, mix together the honey
   and room temperature applesauce.
Apply to cleansed skin with fingertips.
Leave on for 10 minutes.
Rinse.
Apply appropriate moisturizer and sunscreen.

Banana Cream Anti- Acne Mask
Acne and Oily

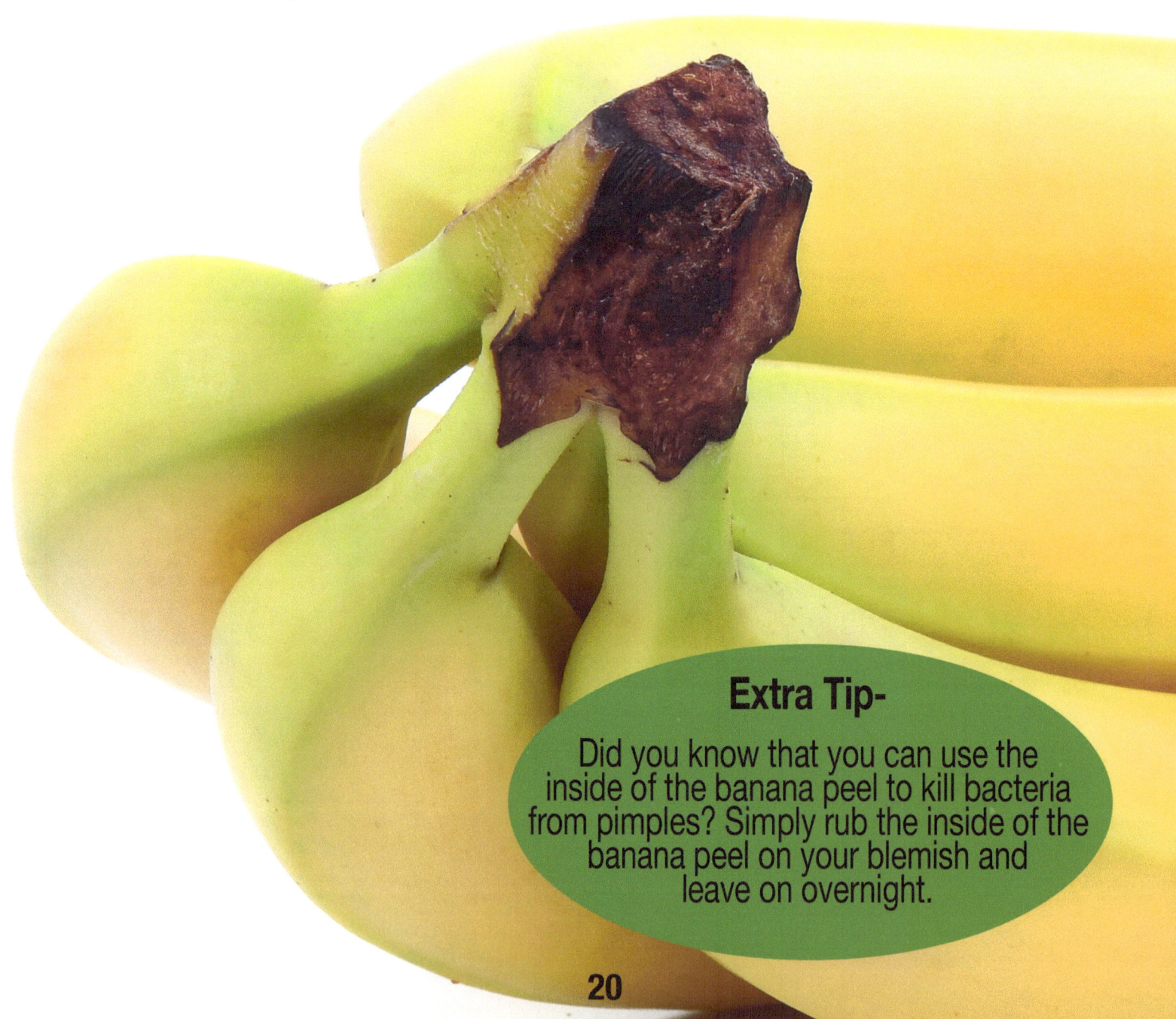

Extra Tip-

Did you know that you can use the inside of the banana peel to kill bacteria from pimples? Simply rub the inside of the banana peel on your blemish and leave on overnight.

20

What You'll Need:

¼ cup of heavy whipping cream
½ small banana
1 Vitamin E capsule

What You'll Do:

Mash banana in a small bowl.
Add cream and mix together to form a paste.
Stir in contents of Vit. E capsule.
Apply over the entire face, neck and décolleté.
Rinse and apply appropriate moisturizer.

Perform 1-2 times a week

Why This Works:

Antioxidants in the banana work to cleanse the skin.
The whipping cream contains lactic acid,
which always helps with blemishes.
The Vitamin E moisturizes and protects the skin.

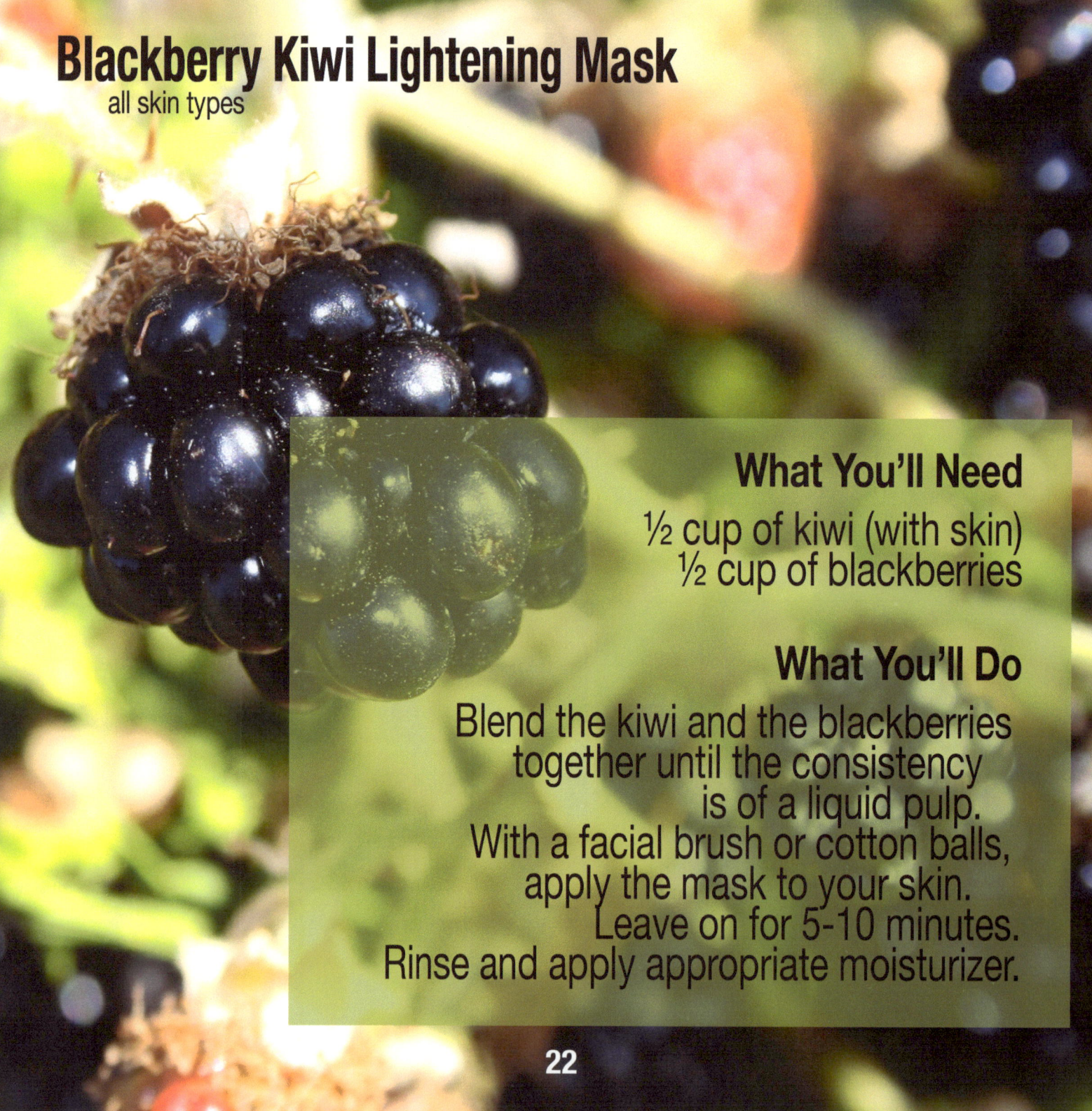

Blackberry Kiwi Lightening Mask
all skin types

What You'll Need
½ cup of kiwi (with skin)
½ cup of blackberries

What You'll Do

Blend the kiwi and the blackberries
together until the consistency
is of a liquid pulp.
With a facial brush or cotton balls,
apply the mask to your skin.
Leave on for 5-10 minutes.
Rinse and apply appropriate moisturizer.

Blueberry Oatmeal Mask

acne-prone skin
oily skin

What You'll Need:

¼ cup of blueberries
¼ cup of oatmeal (the smaller oats)
1 Tablespoon of honey

What You'll Do:

Mash the blueberries with a fork
  (a chunky consistency is ok).
In a small bowl,
  mix the blueberries and oatmeal.
Add the honey.
Apply to cleansed face,
  neck, and décolleté.
Leave on for 10 minutes. Rinse and
  apply appropriate moisturizer
  and sunscreen.

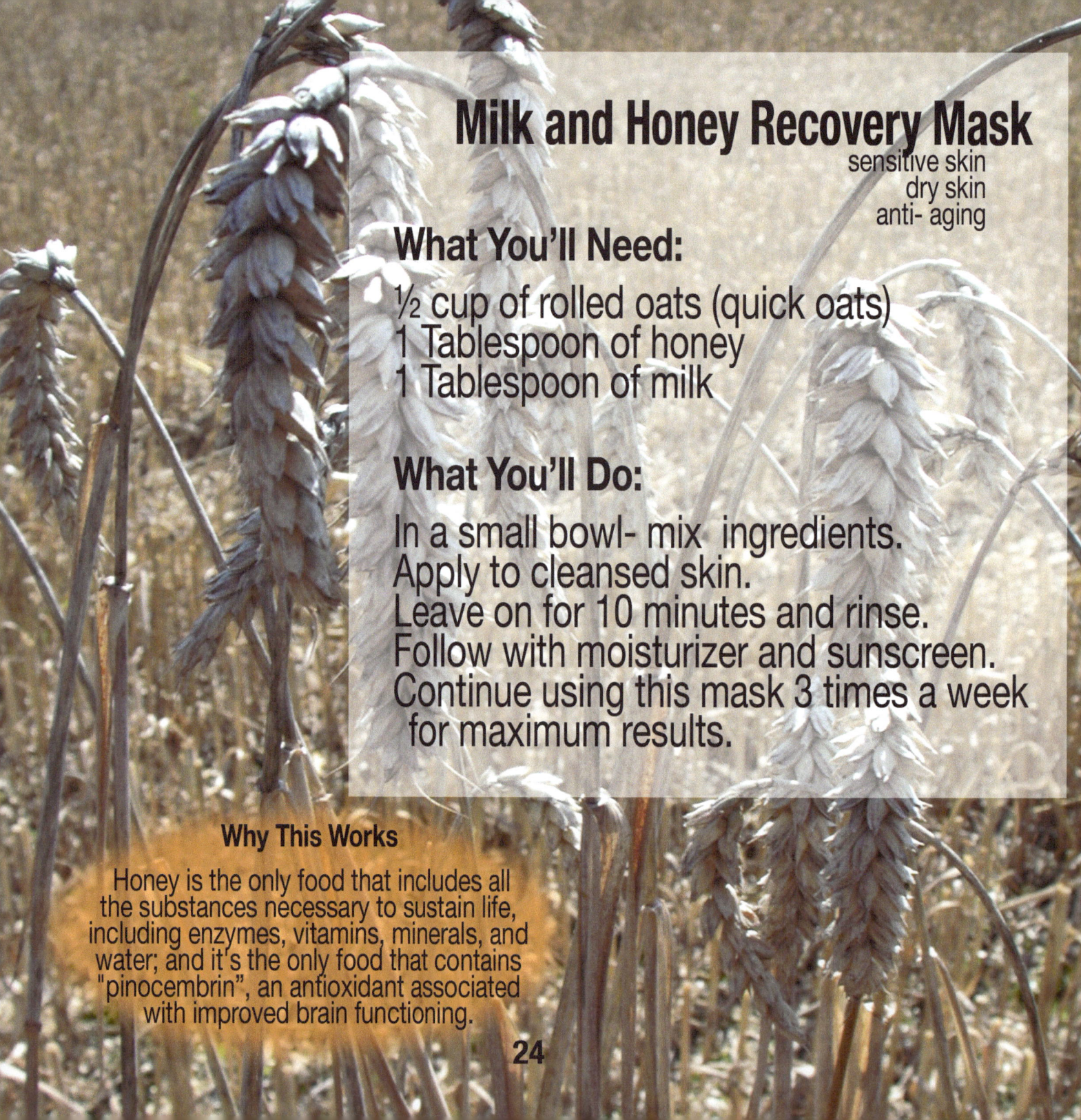

Milk and Honey Recovery Mask

sensitive skin
dry skin
anti- aging

What You'll Need:

½ cup of rolled oats (quick oats)
1 Tablespoon of honey
1 Tablespoon of milk

What You'll Do:

In a small bowl- mix ingredients.
Apply to cleansed skin.
Leave on for 10 minutes and rinse.
Follow with moisturizer and sunscreen.
Continue using this mask 3 times a week
 for maximum results.

Why This Works

Honey is the only food that includes all
the substances necessary to sustain life,
including enzymes, vitamins, minerals, and
water; and it's the only food that contains
"pinocembrin", an antioxidant associated
with improved brain functioning.

24

Yogurt, Cucumber, and Green Tea Comfort Mask

all skin types
great eye mask

What You'll Need:

¼ cucumber- with skin
1 Tablespoon yogurt
1 steeped bag of green tea (warm or cold)

What You'll Do:

Puree cucumber.
In a small bowl, combine the cucumber, yogurt,
    and contents in the tea bag.
Mix together.
Apply to skin, neck, décolleté.
Leave on for 10 minutes.
Rinse.

Avocado Mango Glow

sensitive skin
anti-aging

What You'll Need:
2 Tablespoons of mango
2 Tablespoons of avocado

What You'll Do:
Blend the mango and avocado
   in a blender until you reach
   a smooth consistency.
Apply the mask to cleansed skin.
Leave on for 10 minutes.
Rinse and apply moisturizer and sunscreen.

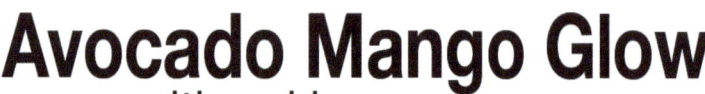

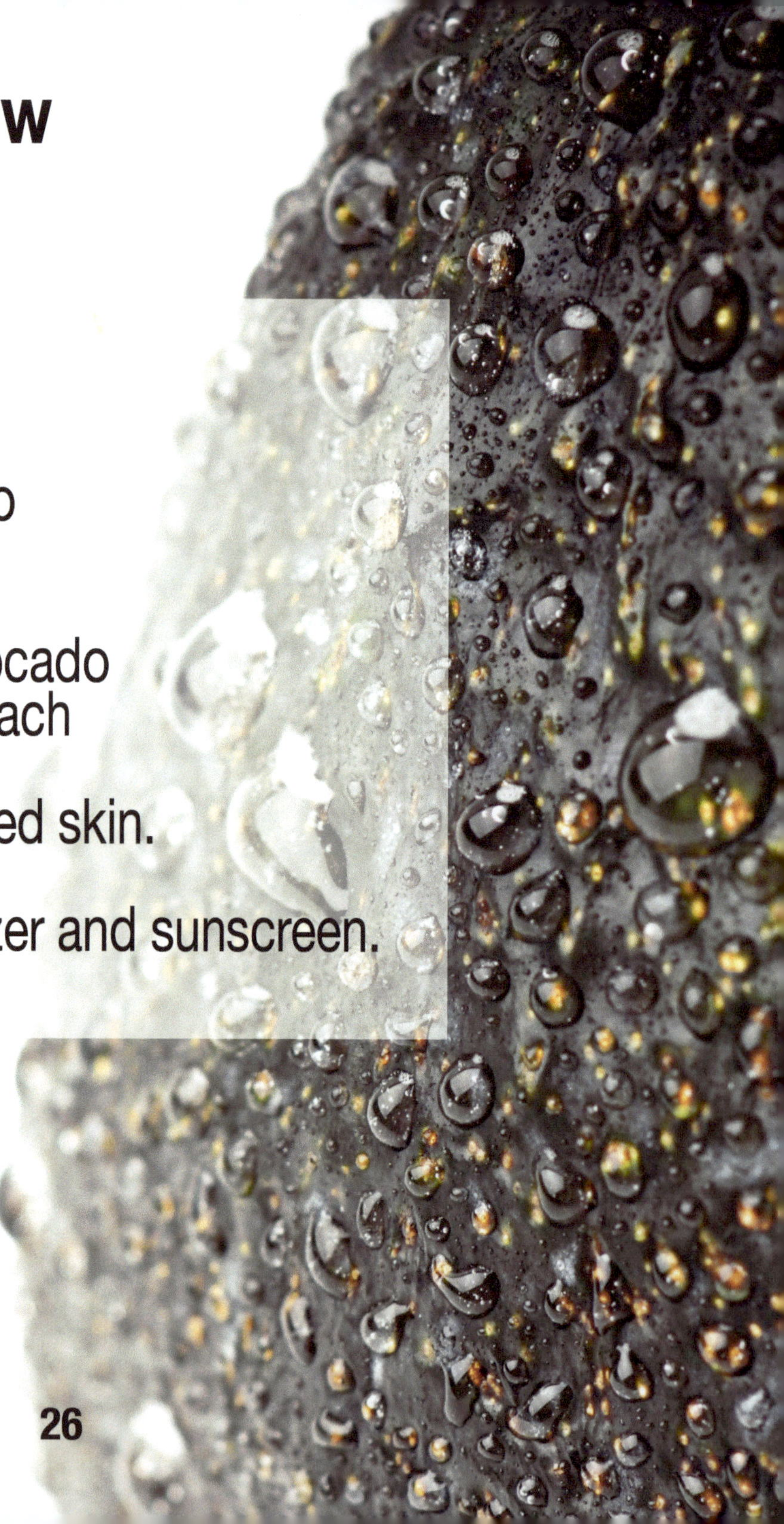

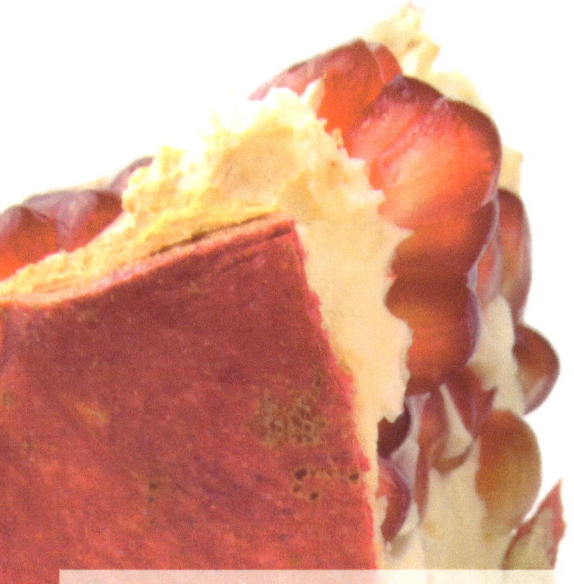

Sweet Potato-Pomegranate Wrinkle Mask

anti-aging
oily
dry

What You'll Need:

¼ cup cooked sweet potatoes
1 Tablespoon of pomegranate seeds
1 teaspoon of honey

What You'll Do:

In a small bowl- mash the pomegranate seeds.
Mix in the other two ingredients.
Apply to face with fingers.
Don't forget the eyes!
Leave on for 10 minutes.
Rinse.
Apply appropriate moisturizer.

27

Smoothie Mask

acne prone
oily skin

What You'll Need:

1 Tablespoon of apple
1 Tablespoon of pear
1 Tablespoon of banana
1 Tablespoon of yogurt

What You'll Do:

Before you begin this fantastic facial mask,
 make sure you mash or blend the three fruits
 until a slightly smooth consistency is obtained.
Be careful that you don't liquefy the fruits,
 a little chunky is okay.
In a small bowl, mix the fruits with the yogurt.
Apply to cleansed skin, face, neck and décolleté.
Rinse after 10 minutes.
Apply appropriate moisturizer and sunscreen.

Kiwi Grapefruit Mask

oily
dry
anti-aging
acne

Spa Tip-

In recent studies,
the scent of grapefruit
makes women appear
to be 10 years younger!
Time to go get some
grapefruit essential oils!

What You'll Need:
½ of a small kiwi
¼ of a grapefruit (juice and pulp)

What You'll Do:
Blend both ingredients
 until consistency is a thick liquid
 (it doesn't need to be smooth).
Apply with cotton balls.
Let it set for 10 minutes- Rinse.
Repeat 2 times a week.

What You'll Need:

2 uncoated aspirin
2 Tablespoons of water
1 Tablespoon of plain yogurt
1 Tablespoon of honey

What You'll Need:

In a small bowl- mix aspirin and water together
  to form a paste.
Add plain yogurt and honey to the aspirin paste.
Apply mask to skin.
Leave on for 5 minutes.
Rinse.

Tip-

This mask works best if applied while taking a shower.
The steam opens the pores,
  which will help the ingredients to penetrate deeper.

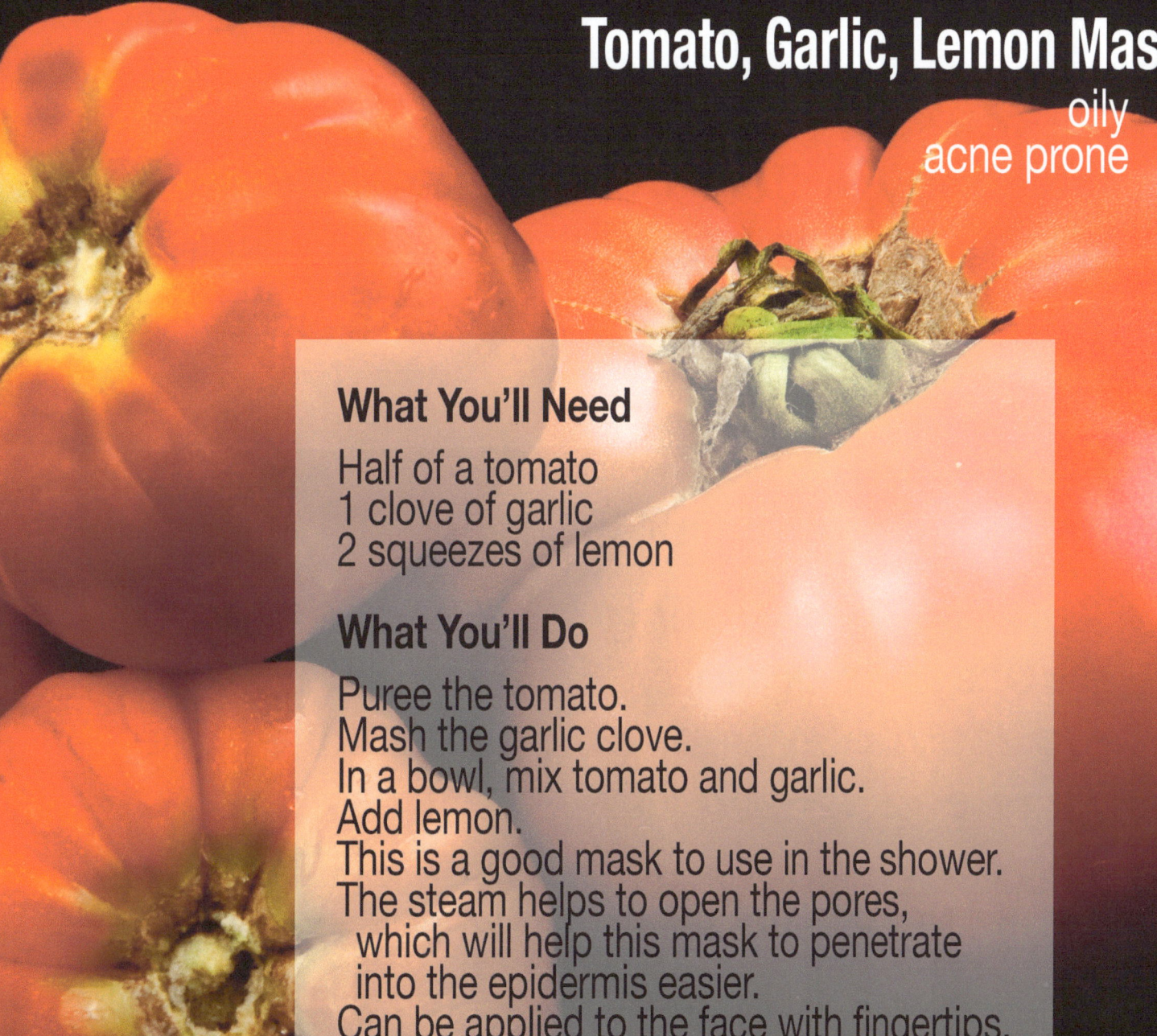

Tomato, Garlic, Lemon Mask

oily
acne prone

What You'll Need

Half of a tomato
1 clove of garlic
2 squeezes of lemon

What You'll Do

Puree the tomato.
Mash the garlic clove.
In a bowl, mix tomato and garlic.
Add lemon.
This is a good mask to use in the shower.
The steam helps to open the pores,
  which will help this mask to penetrate
  into the epidermis easier.
Can be applied to the face with fingertips.
Leave on for a few minutes, then rinse.
Follow with a moisturizer.

31

Body Treatments

Our body suffers from many different skin conditions as well. We deal with rough skin, dehydration, and the inevitable cellulite.

A great way to address those issues is with body treatments.

Two of the following recipes are to exfoliate your body. One is to help reduce the appearance of cellulite. The Seaweed Wrap will help with dehydration. All the recipes will leave your skin feeling silky smooth!

Take note- these could be messy! Just follow the instructions. For best results, do a treatment once a week for 6 weeks.

Chocolate Covered Strawberry Scrub

body treatment

What You'll Need:
½ cup of pureed or blended strawberries
¼ cup of cocoa
½ cup of sugar
1 Tablespoon of cream

What You'll Do:
In a medium bowl, mix all of the ingredients together.
While in the shower or bath,
    rub contents over entire body,
    scrubbing in circular motions.
 Rinse.
Apply body lotion.
Can be done once or twice a week.

33

Pumpkin Pie Body Scrub
body treatment

What You'll Need:

1 cup of mashed pumpkin (canned is ok)
1 cup of brown sugar (light or dark)
1 teaspoon of cinnamon

What You'll Do:

In a medium bowl, mix together all three ingredients.
Take in the shower and apply scrub over entire body,
  scrubbing until the brown sugar dissolves.
Make sure you scrub on the rough areas
  (knees, elbows, etc.).
Rinse while in shower.
Your skin will feel incredibly smooth.
This can be done once a week.

Café Mocha Latte Cellulite Scrub
body treatment

What You'll Need:

1 cup of used, caffeinated coffee grounds
½ cup of milk
1 Tablespoon of cocoa
Dash of cinnamon

What You'll Do:

In a medium bowl, mix all four ingredients together.
Take mixture to shower. While in the shower,
scrub the entire body. Paying special attention
to the troubled cellulite areas, scrub in circular motions
for about a minute. Rinse. Do this a couple times
a week for maximum results.
Please note- this could be messy!

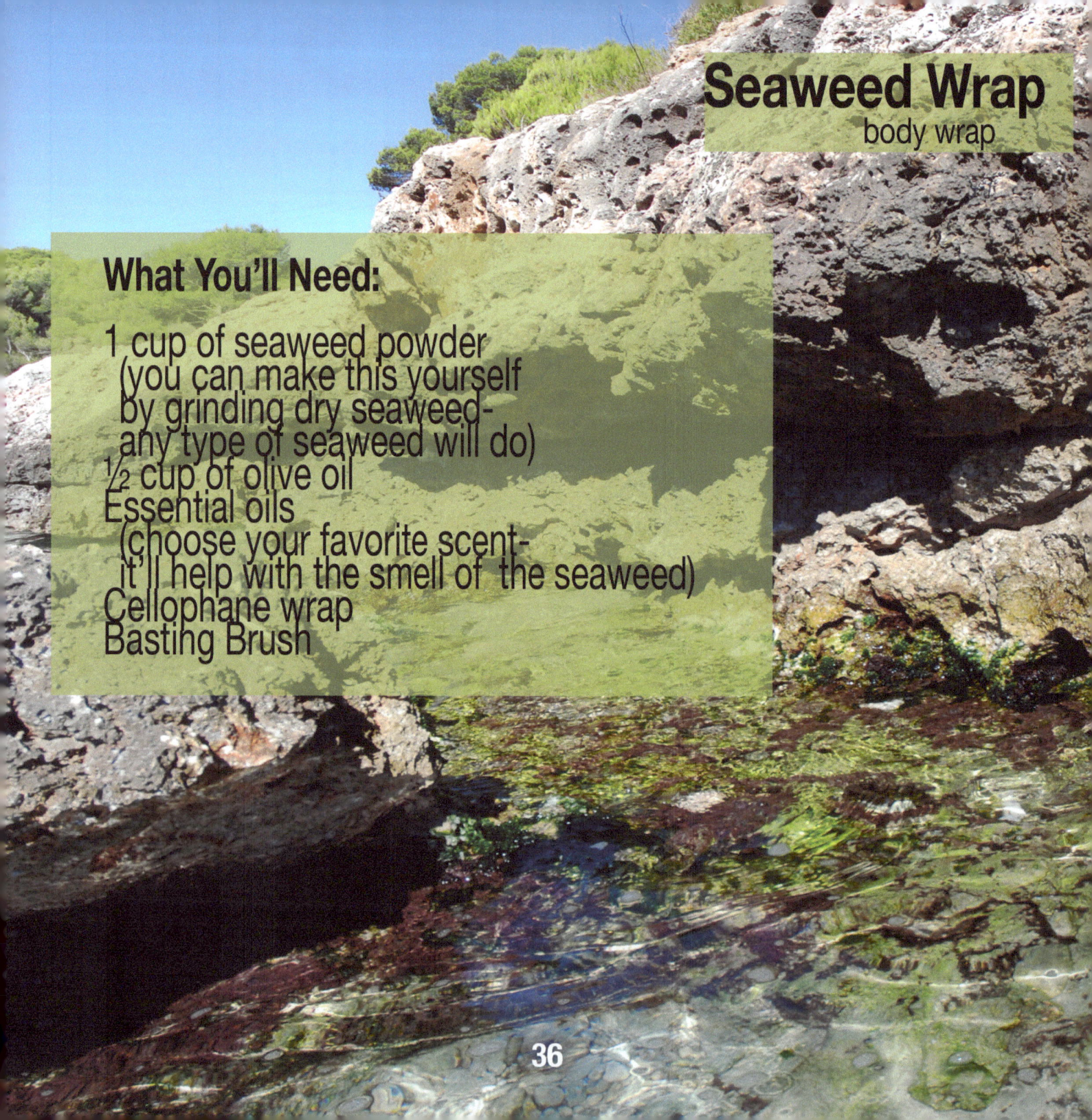

Seaweed Wrap
body wrap

What You'll Need:

1 cup of seaweed powder
  (you can make this yourself
  by grinding dry seaweed-
  any type of seaweed will do)
½ cup of olive oil
Essential oils
  (choose your favorite scent-
  it'll help with the smell of the seaweed)
Cellophane wrap
Basting Brush

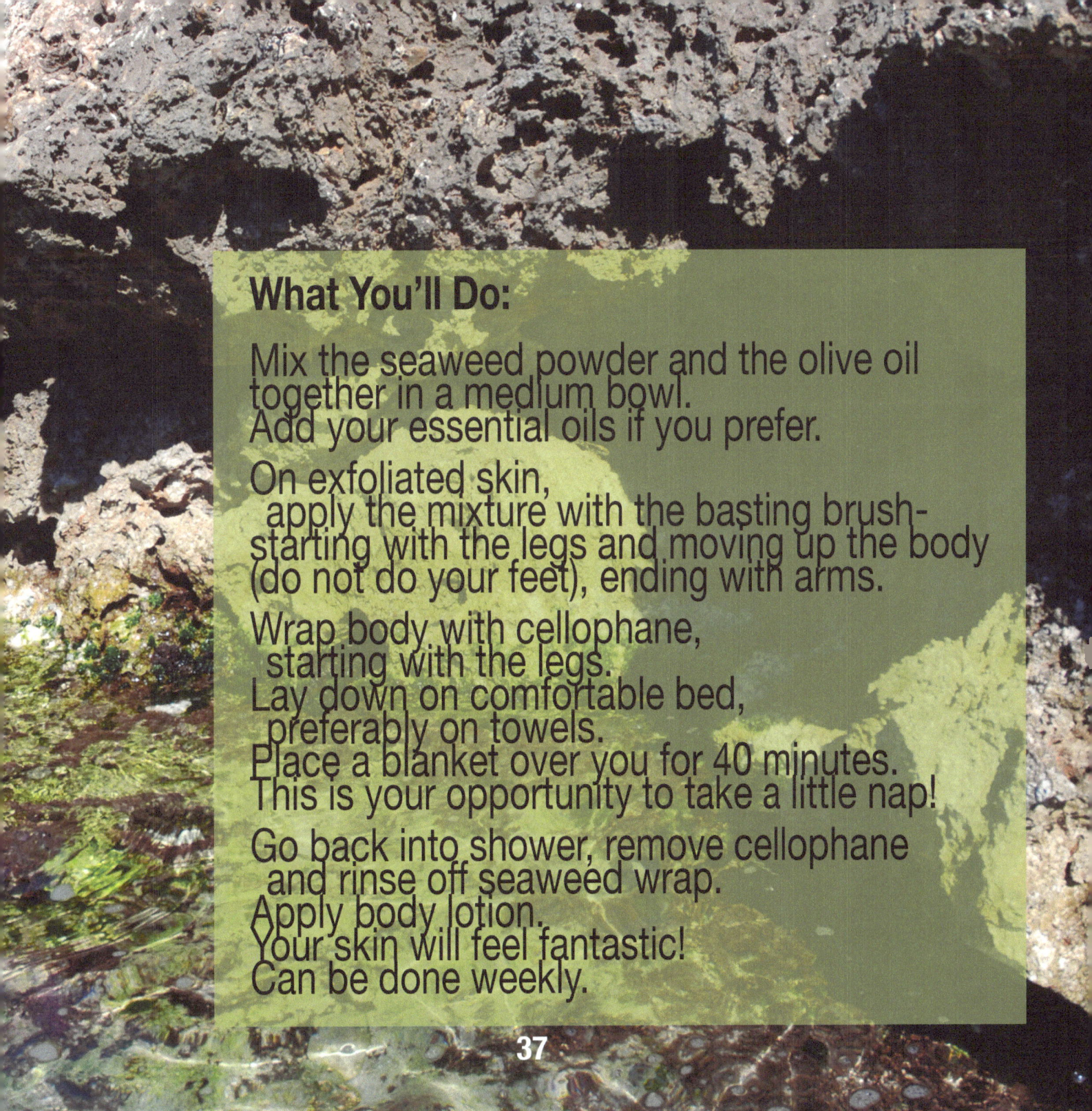

What You'll Do:

Mix the seaweed powder and the olive oil
together in a medium bowl.
Add your essential oils if you prefer.

On exfoliated skin,
 apply the mixture with the basting brush-
starting with the legs and moving up the body
(do not do your feet), ending with arms.

Wrap body with cellophane,
 starting with the legs.
Lay down on comfortable bed,
 preferably on towels.
Place a blanket over you for 40 minutes.
This is your opportunity to take a little nap!

Go back into shower, remove cellophane
 and rinse off seaweed wrap.
Apply body lotion.
Your skin will feel fantastic!
Can be done weekly.

Special Acknowledgement

I personally want to thank Betsy Kortebein who created the graphics for this book.
She has taught me that if you mentally challenge yourself, the physical ability will follow, not only in health, but in life.

Betsy, you're a true inspiration to me and so many others.   -DeeDee

Betsy Kortebein

Betsy got her Design degree from UCLA while teaching fitness classes, as a part time job. She feels fortunateto have continued with both careers throughout the years.

www.ingramcontent.com/pod-product-compliance
Lightning Source LLC
Chambersburg PA
CBHW041520280526

45792CB00004B/1324